Sugar Detox Diet:

Effective Methods To Become Healthier And Happier Without Sugar in Three Weeks

The information herein is offered for informational purposes solely, and is universal as so. The presentation of the information is without contract or any type of guarantee assurance.

The trademarks that are used are without any consent, and the publication of the trademark is without permission or backing by the trademark owner. All trademarks and brands within this book are for clarifying purposes only and are the owned by the owners themselves, not affiliated with this document.

Table of content

Introduction

Sugar was first introduced into western diets in the 11th Century; it was a result of the Crusades. Until then sugar had been a 'spice' used only by Arab and African countries.

This first taste of sugar led to an explosion in demand. In 1319 AD sugar was available in London at a rate which would today equate to USD 100 per kilo! Fortunately, it has come down significantly in price and is now available in virtually every shop you enter.

Unfortunately, sugar is addictive, although not in the same way as drugs such as heroin. Drugs create a physical dependency in the body; without which you cannot function properly.

Sugar, on the other hand, creates the same neurologically responses as these highly addictive drugs. You will experience heightened pleasure, a burst of energy and a desire for more; but only because it is pleasurable; not because the body needs it.

This pleasure is caused by the release of opioids and dopamine; the more sugar you consume the more your body will crave this feeling. You will need to continually eat more sugar to gain the same feeling; even though you know it will have a detrimental effect on your health.

It may not be classed as addictive in the same way that heroin is, but the results are similar. But, because this is not seen as an issue and sugar is in virtually every food item; it s not actually seen as an issue!

The fact of the matter is that science has shown sugar to be linked to a variety of detrimental health conditions:

- **Weight Gain**

Sugar is a valuable source of energy for the human body. However, if you consume more calories than you need, your body will store the excess as fat. The more sugar you eat the more likely it is that you will gain weight.

- **Tooth Decay**

The consumption of sugar is proven to cause increased levels of tooth decay. Sugar sticks to your teeth and attacks the enamel coating; weakening your tooth and allowing it to decay much faster than it would naturally.

Bad teeth can lead to a host of other issues; including blood infections.

- **Heart Disease**

This is actually connected to the fact that excess sugar causes a fat build up in your body. This fatty substance will not just sit on your organs making it harder for them to do their job. It will also start to clog up your blood vessels; restricting blood flow round your body and leading to muscle wastage.

The heart is a muscle and can experience muscle wastage; the result is heart disease and even death.

- **Diabetes**

You are probably already aware that diabetes is the result of your body being unable to produce insulin in sufficient quantities to deal with the sugar in your blood.

Unfortunately, this condition is often brought about by excessive sugar consumption and being overweight.

- **Mood Swings & Headaches**

Sugar gives you a burst of energy and a natural high. Unfortunately this is followed by a low. This is often seen in children but is actually relevant in all walks of life.

Feeling great then feeling down is the initial stages of mood swings; which will become worse as you continue to consume excessive amounts of sugar.

The mood swings and fluctuation in hormones can often lead to headaches as your body struggles to adapt to a rapidly changing environment.

- **Immune System Issues**

Finally, excess sugar consumption has been linked with immune system issues.

Research is still ongoing into this side effect of sugar but the current studies show that increased levels of sugar in your body will increase the amount of bacteria and yeast in your body; they feed on the sugar.

This increase will knock your immune system off-balance and make you more prone to illness.

Chapter 1 – Ditching the Sugar

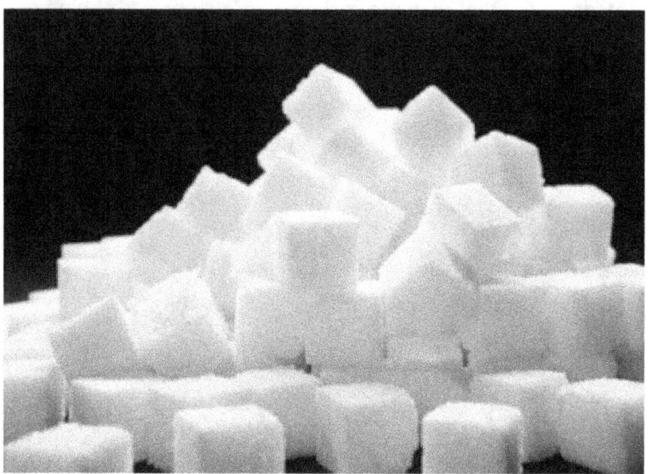

https://timedotcom.files.wordpress.com/2015/10/sugar.jpg?w=720

There is no doubt that sugar is of use to the body; it is a fast source of energy; as opposed to carbohydrates which are a slower burning fuel. It is not the consumption of sugar which is the issue; it is the excess consumption and the fact that you will constantly want more.

It is this realization that brings many people to consider the sugar detox. If you have any doubt regarding sugar's responsibility for the current levels of obesity then you should consider the fact that current statistics show the average American is consuming 28KG of sugar a year; just through sugar added to products you purchase in shops.

Current estimates suggest sugar is responsible for 14 % of your daily calorific intake; the target should be just 5%!

However, between the addiction that is created and the level of sugar found in everyday food items; it is very difficult to remove sugar completely from your diet. The idea of going 'cold turkey' is not necessarily an appealing one, but, as with many addictions; it is the most effective way to relieve an addiction and become both healthier and happier.

It is important to note that natural sugars are not an issue; it is the sugars that are added to food that you need to avoid. To start your detox you need to learn the following lessons:

1. Mental Preparation

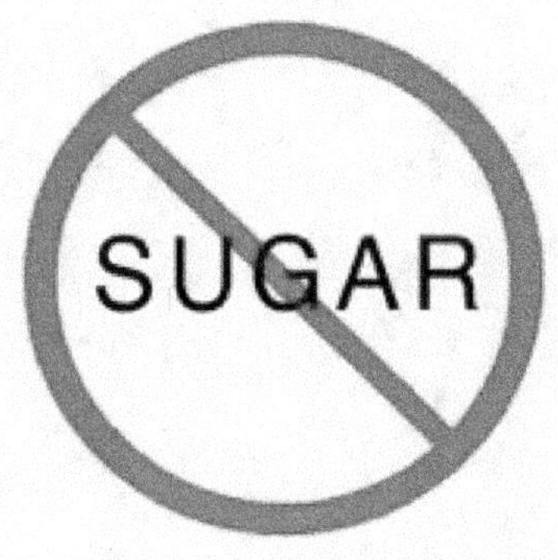

As with any addiction you must first accept that you have an issue. You may already be aware of this and be ready to do something about it; this is good!

If not, then your first step must be to realize you have an issue; as many people do. You can accept this issue through the following methods:

> Taking an obesity or even diabetic quiz online to find out if you are at risk of diabetes and considered obese or overweight.

> Speak to others who have already completed a sugar detox and consider their opinions.

> Make a food diary to show what you are actually eating; your sugar dependency will become obvious once you evaluate which foods have added sugar in them.

> Review your current health. Consuming excess sugar does more than cause weight gain. It can be the reason you are tired all the time, have memory issues or suffer from sinus issues.

Once you have completed one (or all) of these quizzes you will see that you have a problem with sugar.

You must accept the issue and be determined to do something about it; for your own sake. This is important as your motivation is what will get you through the difficult withdrawal phase.

2. Cold Turkey

As mentioned, cold turkey is the way forward; no matter how difficult it may seem. This period can be difficult and you are best to enlist a loved one to give you some support.

Part of the process can take two weeks, depending upon your level of addiction, but the results will be worth it.

To go cold turkey you should eliminate all products in your house which have added sugar in them. This includes sweetened soft drinks.

The most effective way to do this is to avoid anything which comes in a can or packet with a label and more than one ingredient. It is also advisable to give up all grains for the two weeks; this will prevent your metabolism from slowing or your cravings from getting worse.

3. **Drink**

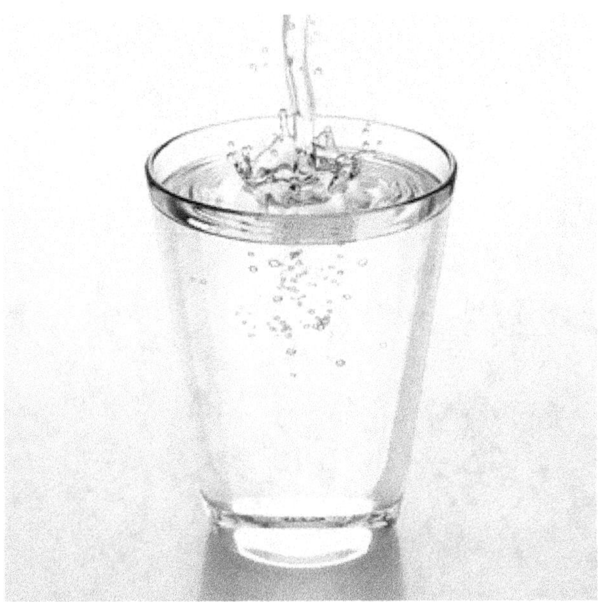

http://assets.goodhousekeeping.co.uk/main/embedded/25836/glass_water__large.jpg?20150721154507

The best thing you can drink is water. This will help your body to flush out toxins and overcome the cravings.

It is also important to note that any drink which has sugar in it will go straight to your liver where the sugar will be turned into fat. Consuming liquid sugar is inviting fat growth; especially on your belly.

Alongside water it is safe to drink green tea, black coffee and almost any other drink that does not have added sugar and that you do not add sugar to.

4. Protein and Carbohydrates

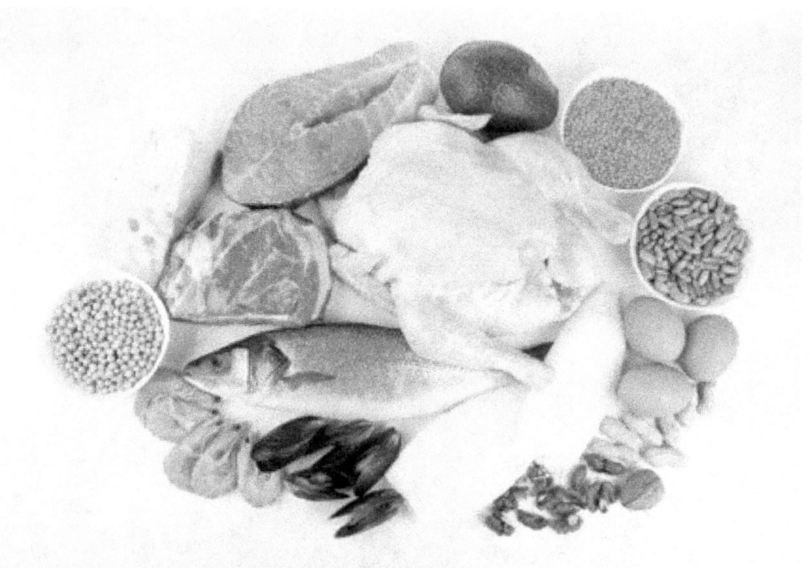

http://www.leanandmuscular.org/resources/shutterstock_233300935.jpg

Protein is essential for building muscles and repairing cells. However, what you may not know is that it also plays an important part in balancing the hormones in the body; particularly blood sugar and insulin.

Carbohydrates are your energy. Instead of a quick burst as delivered by a sugar hit, carbohydrates will supply you with a slow release of energy over a long period of time. This ensures your energy levels remain consistent throughout the day and avoids the crash after sugar consumption.

There is no limit to the amount of carbs you can eat, although it is advisable to leave potatoes, sweet potatoes and winter squash out of your detox diet.

5. Consume Fat

Your goal is to beat an addiction to sugar but in the process you will need to learn to eat healthier and you will lose weight.

Fat is one of the issues which is often misunderstood. Fat is actually an essential part of your diet; it can help to keep you feeling full, balance your blood cells and even be used as energy. There are good fats and bad fats; you should concentrate on consuming the good ones, which can be found in abundance in products such as nuts, olive oil and avocados.

6. Sugar Snacks

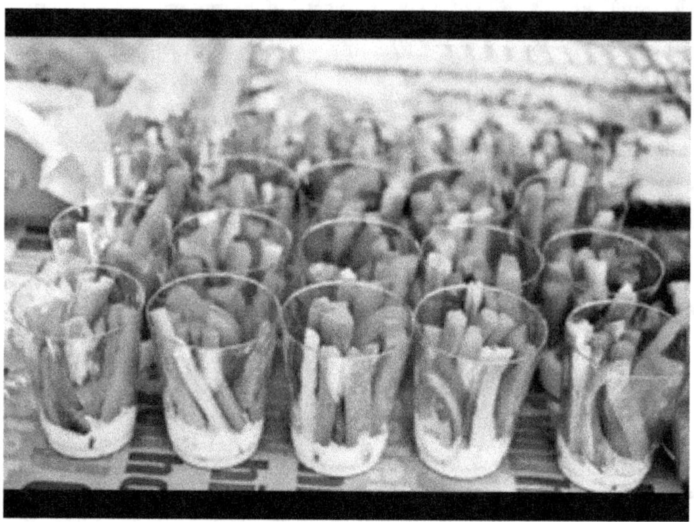

https://i.ytimg.com/vi/oF0tEo1xaow/hqdefault.jpg

When you detox your body is trying to rebalance its hormones and learn to live without sugar. This means that there will be moments when the balance is not correct and your blood sugar level will drop.

You will crave sugar. Fortunately, unlike a recovering drug addict you can actually indulge in sugar; but only natural ones.

To be ready for these cravings you must have a selection of healthy sugar snacks on hand. This can include a packet of nuts, meat jerky or salmon jerky, or even some fruit.

This will introduce natural sugars into your body, quickly restoring the balance without resorting to the artificial, added sugars.

7. **Monitor Stress**

Stress can play havoc with your body. When you are stressed your body produces cortisol, ready to either fight or flight. Unfortunately your body will want to fuel the need to flight and will immediately crave a sugar boost to provide instantly usable energy.

Of course, when you do not respond with flight as you are dealing with a stressful situation at work, your body simply stores the sugar you consumed as more body fat.

You need to avoid stressful situations wherever possible. You can also negate the effects of the cortisol by taking several deep breathes. These must be done slowly, allowing the body to calm and the craving to pass.

8. **Sleep**

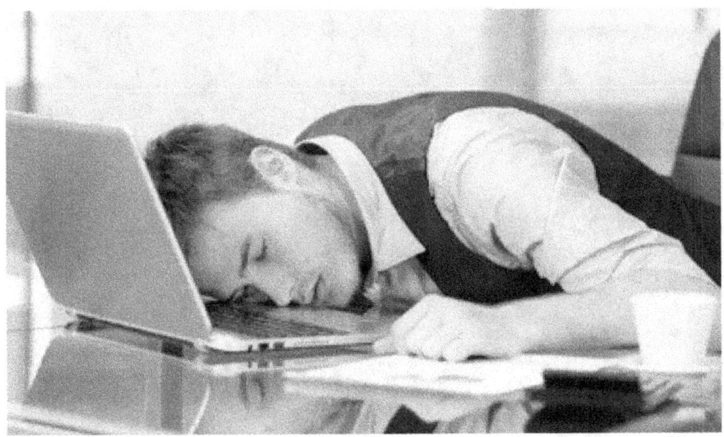

http://www.helpguide.org/images/sleep/man-sleeping-on-desk-500.jpg

Sleep is actually an essential part of being healthy. It doesn't matter if you feel great on just 2 hours sleep a night. Your body needs a minimum of 5 hours sleep, preferably between 6 and 8.

Sleep allows your body to regulate its hormones. During this time the levels of hunger hormones decrease and appetite suppressing hormones increase. If you do not get enough sleep these hormones are not suppressed and you will feel hungry as soon as you wake.

The lack of sleep will mean that you need an energy boost and your first thought will be a sugar laden snack.

Now that you are armed with the right information you are ready to go 'cold turkey'. However, it is worth noting that once you make this decision you need to commit to it straight away; there is no point saying you will start the detox next week.

Chapter 2 – How To Live Without Sugar

Getting yourself in the right mind set and clearing the added sugar products from your home will help you get off to a good start. But, you will need more than that in order to achieve your goal.

You now need to learn how to live without sugar. This means finding alternatives to sugar laden products. The following lessons will help you to achieve this aim and teach you what to eat in the future.

Foods to Avoid

> **Fruit & Dairy**

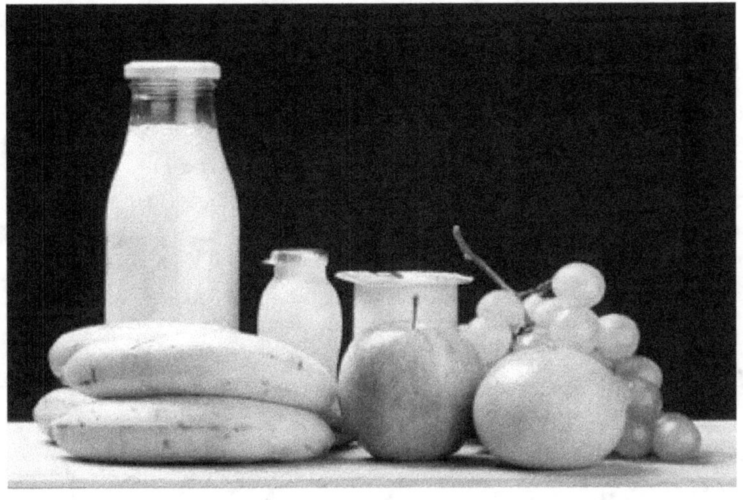

https://www.camelbackvending.com/wp-content/uploads/2012/10/bigstock-Dairy-And-Fruit-24954521.jpg

These are actually healthy foods which have naturally sugars in; providing they do not say 'added sugar' on the label. However, for the first 5 days of your sugar detox you should try to avoid these items.

The reason for this is that the natural sugars will interfere with your ability to cut sugar completely. It is better to stop all sugar and then re-introduce the healthy ones than it is to attempt to separate them for your detox.

➢ Flour Products

As mentioned already, flour also needs to be stopped for the first few days of your detox. Flour is a refined carb which contains starch, a substance which has been linked with sugar addiction; it is advisable to stop using it for the duration of your detox; allowing your body to withdraw cleanly.

This can be the most challenging part as even home cooking often requires flour.

➢ Drinks

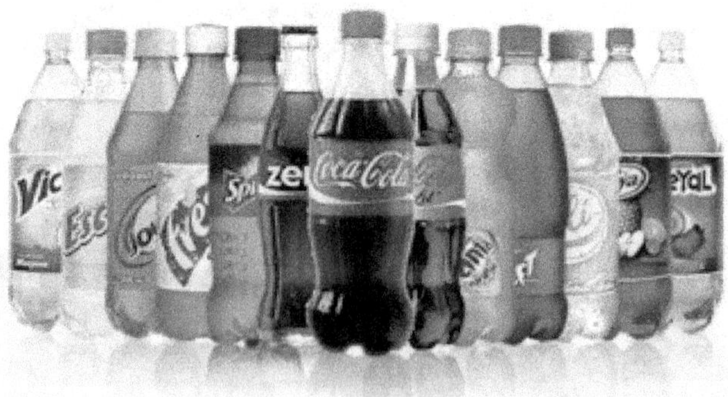

Your regular coffee will need to be replaced for the duration of the detox. You should focus on water, one black coffee a day and as much green or herbal tea as you like. You should not have any soft drinks, whether they are sweetened naturally or artificially.

➢ Alcohol

All alcohol should be avoided as many drinks are made through a yeast process which encourages sugar addiction. Other drinks are actually made with, or sweetened by sugar.

Skipping alcohol can also give your body a respite and a chance to rebuild itself.

➢ Processed Meats

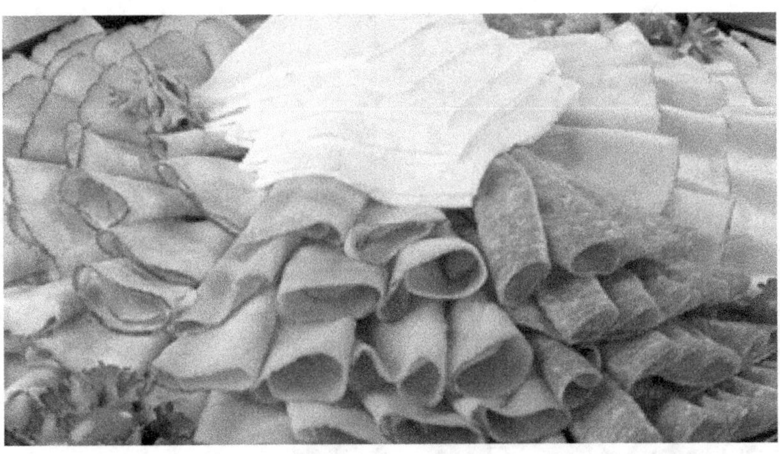

http://www.france-surgery.com/wp-content/uploads/2015/10/processed-meat-early-death.jpg

The majority of processed food has sugar added to make it taste sweeter and leave you wanting more of it. This is why it is important to eliminate all processed foods from your diet during your sugar detox.

You may re-introduce them after the detox but you must be aware of how much sugar is in them and the level you should be consuming.

➢ Sauces

Almost all sauces have a high sugar content. This is for the same reasons as the processed food; building your addiction and not helping you.

Avoid all sauces for the duration of your detox, you will probably find that you do not want them after the detox is over!

➢ Sweets

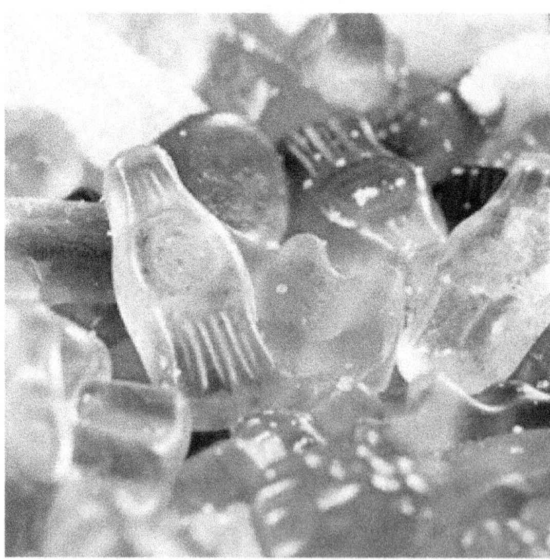

Finally, it should be fairly obvious but all sweet items are off the menu! Ant shop created sweet treat will be stuffed full of sugar. You cannot afford to give into temptation on this one!

Now that you have eliminated the danger foods from your home you should stock up on the foods you need to eat while on your sugar detox.

- **Non-Processed Meat**

- **Vegetables**

- **Fish**

- **Eggs**

- **Olive Oil**

- **Nuts & Seeds**

- **Corn**

- **Quinoa**

- **Brown Rice**

These food types can all be consumed in abundance as they do not have any sugar in them.

An example of one day's worth of meals could be:

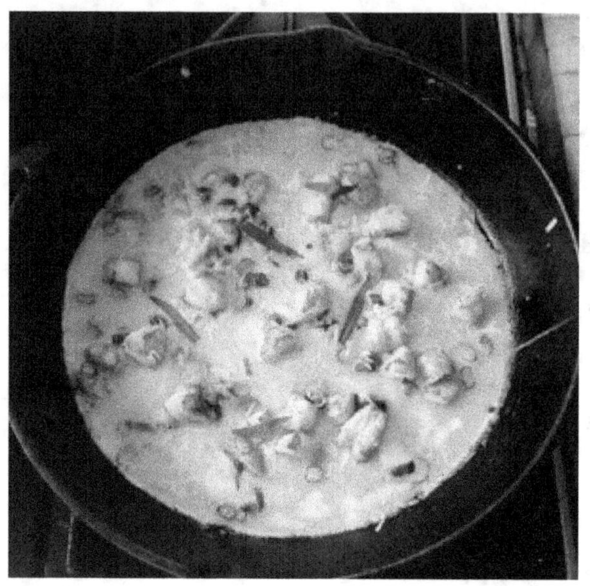

https://static1.squarespace.com/static/535ae385e4b0153c8b58e24f/t/5411eea6e4b0c978ce0925cd/1410461359612/

Breakfast – Omelet with shrimp and tarragon

Lunch – Fresh turkey meat grilled with salad, mushrooms and kale chips.

Dinner – Baked fish of your choice with brown rice and green beans

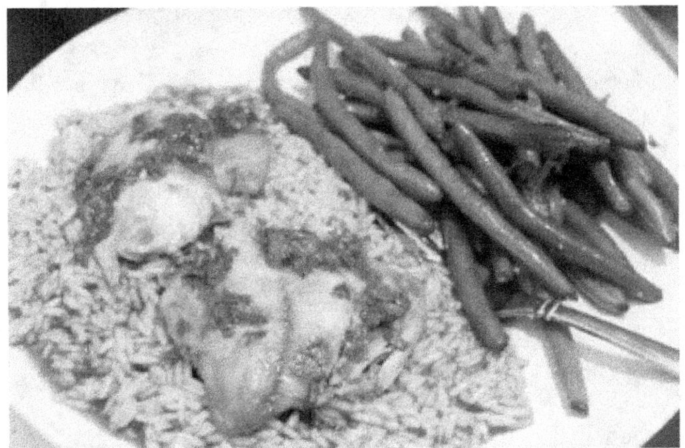

https://seehatsie.files.wordpress.com/2012/05/6cc2d-img_1205.jpg

Snacks throughout the day can be nuts or sliced pepper; if required.

By changing the meat and the salad / vegetables with each dish it is possible to create a week's worth of meals in no time!

Half way through your detox you can start to bring back in some of the items which have natural sugars; these include:

- **Fruit**

- **Dark Chocolate** – as long as it is 100%

- **Dairy Products** – Introduce these slowly to prevent an issue with sugar or any dairy intolerance.

- **Wine** – This should only be added in small amounts

- **Whole grain foods** - including pasta and bread.

There are several reasons why it is important to re-introduce foods into your diet half way through the detox and not at the end.

Your Palate

Once you have completed the sugar detox for a week you will have managed to wipe your palate; your body will have gone through the worst f the withdrawal and you will be ready to really taste food again.

Foods which before the detox were sour will now be much sweeter. Your palate will be recalibrated for the future!

- **Interest**

It can be difficult to stick to any diet which limits your food choices. By introducing some of the foods that you will be eating long term you will keep your interest and focus on the detox.

You will also be building your lifestyle choices regarding how you will approach food in the future.

- **Health benefits**

Undertaking a sugar detox is to reduce or eliminate your body's dependency on artificial sugar. It is not designed to make you suffer but to offer a range of health benefits.

There are those that say the detox can be completed quicker, but the two approaches will allow you to detox and slowly rebuild your diet without having the unnecessary pressure of a 3 day detox.

Completing the detox is only the first stage of your journey! You are now learning about the different sugars available and that some are essential for your continued good health.

There are three important lessons to learn whilst completing a sugar detox:

1. Know Your Sugar Limits

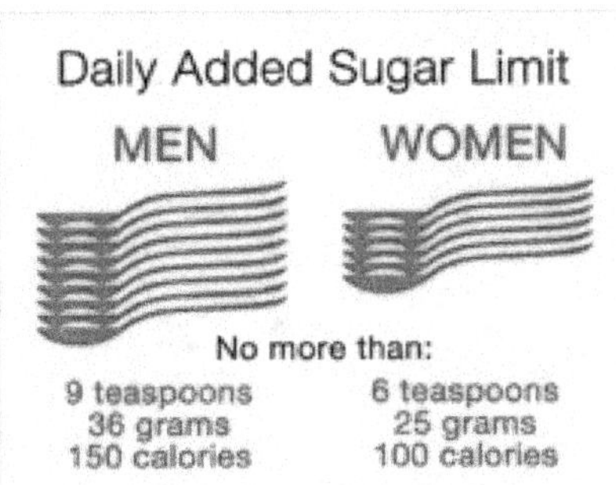

http://www.heart.org/idc/groups/heart-public/@wcm/@fc/documents/image/~extract/UCM_470043~5~staticrendition/medium.jpg

The average male adult should consume a maximum of 36g of sugar a day. This is the equivalent of 9 sugar cubes! Women should limit their sugar intake to 25g per day; or 6 teaspoons.

Children under 6 should have no more than 19g while those between 7 and 10 can have 24g a day.

Children under 4 should not have any product with added sugar

It is important to note that the above guidelines apply to what is referred to as 'free sugars'. These are artificial sugars. Sugar found naturally in dairy products, fruit and other foods do not count as part of your sugar intake.

It is also recommended that no more than 5% of your calorie intake per day comes from free sugars.

2. Understanding Free Sugars

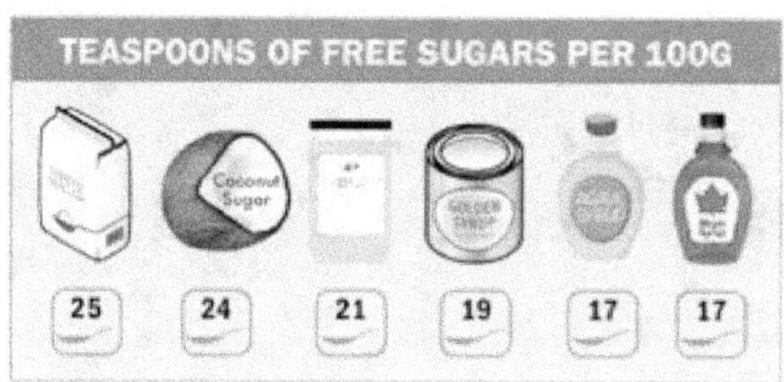

http://sugarfreelondoner.com/wp-content/uploads/2017/07/Screen-Shot-2017-07-21-at-18.17.02.png

Free sugars are those which are added to food. You can find them in soft drinks, biscuits, chocolate, flavored yoghurts and cereal. In fact, they can appear in almost any item which has been created by a manufacturer!

Natural sugars do not generally count as free sugar with the exception of those found in honey, syrups and unsweetened fruit juices.

Free sugars are the ones which are deemed to be bad for your health and lead to weight gain, as well as other health issues.

3. The Role of Sugar in Your Body

Sugar is essential to your body. It provides you with energy. Carbohydrates also provide energy but they release the energy slowly. Sugar creates instant energy but it can also be stored and it is known to be beneficial to retaining muscle mass.

This is why it is important to have sugar in your diet, but, where possible to stay away from free sugars and stick to natural ones.

Consuming sugar is also important because if you do not have enough sugar in your body then your muscles will start to burn protein instead.

While this may seem beneficial, it is in fact removing protein from your muscles and other organs which need it. Prolonged low sugar levels will lead to a decrease in muscle mass unless you consume a large amount of additional protein.

It is also worth noting that your body is capable of converting glucose into amino acids to help fulfill the needs of your body.

Chapter 3 – Health Benefits Offered Within 3 Weeks

A sugar detox will provide you with a range of benefits that are sure to leave you feeling happier and healthier within 3 weeks. In general the detox will be completed in 2, the extra week will provide you with a chance to evaluate the success of the detox and establish your new, healthier eating habits.

These benefits are shown in this chapter, but you should also have learned the following lessons:

- **Sugar is Everywhere**

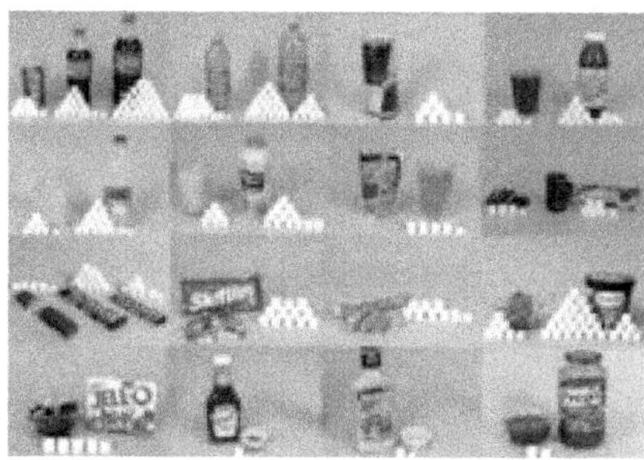

https://i2.wp.com/www.healthyplatesmnt.com/wp-content/uploads/2015/03/too-much-sugar1.jpg?resize=296%2C209

By now it should be abundantly clear that sugar is in practically everything you eat. The difference is in selecting foods which have plenty of natural sugars and avoiding those with added sugar.

It is very difficult to count the exact amount of sugar you are consuming which is why it is so important to consume only natural sugars. These are classified as simple sugars and can be used by the body in a variety of ways.

- **Take Time When Choosing and Eating Food**

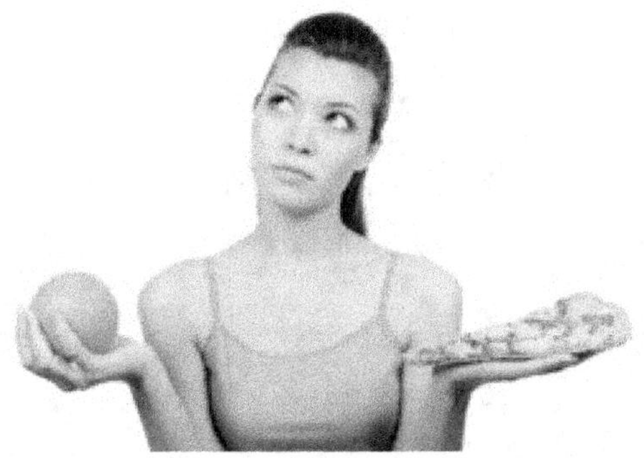

https://beautyhealthtips.in/wp-content/uploads/2014/08/How-to-choose-right-food-for-health.jpg

Completing a sugar detox means having to think about the food you will be eating and the content of the food you normally buy. This is a great opportunity to improve your food choices and become more aware of everything that is in your food; not just the level of sugar.

Slowing down the process of choosing and preparing food will help to ensure your choices are healthier and your food is actually more enjoyable.

- **Protein Helps**

Removing sugar from your diet is likely to have two effects. The first is that you will crave sugar. Your body has become used to consuming large quantities of sugar; the sudden change in diet will leave you obsessing about sugar!

To minimize these cravings you must consume more protein; particularly at breakfast and lunch.

The second effect is a lack of energy later in the day. This is common for many people as you will be watching what you eat. While this is a good thing, you will be likely to avoid simply replacing sugar with carbs as the detox steers you away from carbs in general.

However, carb intake is essential to maintain your energy levels; reducing carb and sugar intake is likely to leave you without enough calories to reach your maintenance level; the result is you will feel tired and sluggish later in the day.

- **You Will Have Bad days**

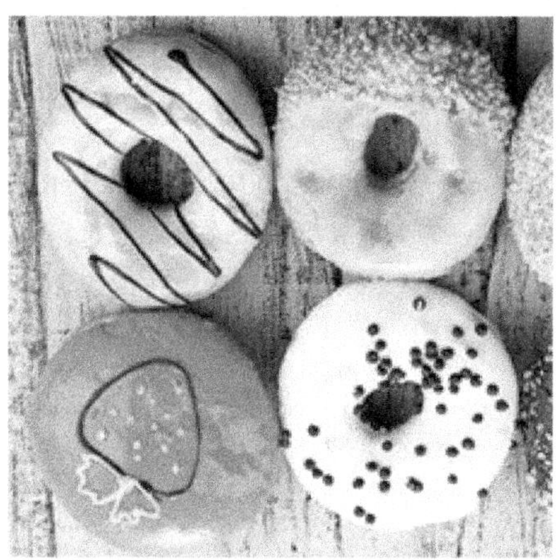

http://global-cdn.skinnyms.com/wp-content/uploads/2015/05/7-Day-Sugar-Detox-Thumbnail.jpg

Any form of cold turkey is hard work; regardless of what substance you are withdrawing from.

Your body will crave sugar and you are likely to have headaches, be irritable and have other withdrawal symptoms.

You need to accept that there will be difficult times and temptation. This is when you will need the support of your loved ones to focus on your goal.

- **High Sugar Consumption is Linked to Health Issues**

High levels of sugar in your diet are linked with weight gain and the destruction of your teeth. But, you are also increasing your risk of diabetes, heart disease and some types of cancer.

A sugar detox will allow you to minimize or even eliminate your consumption of sugar and improve your overall health in the process.

- **Ditching Sugar Does Not equate to Instant Weight Loss**

Removing sugar from your diet reduces the number of calories you are consuming. However, a lower calorie intake does not always equate to weight loss.

To lose weight you need to consume fewer calories than your body needs to on a daily basis. Removing sugar may not be enough to put you below your required calorie intake each day.

This is not a bad thing! Your body should only undertake one of these types of challenges at a time. If your aim is to lose weight then complete the sugar detox first and then start considering your calorie intake and the level of exercise you need to do.

The Benefits of a Sugar Detox

There is no doubt that a sugar detox will provide you with a range of health benefits. Completing the challenge may be difficult but the results are worthwhile:

1. **Health**

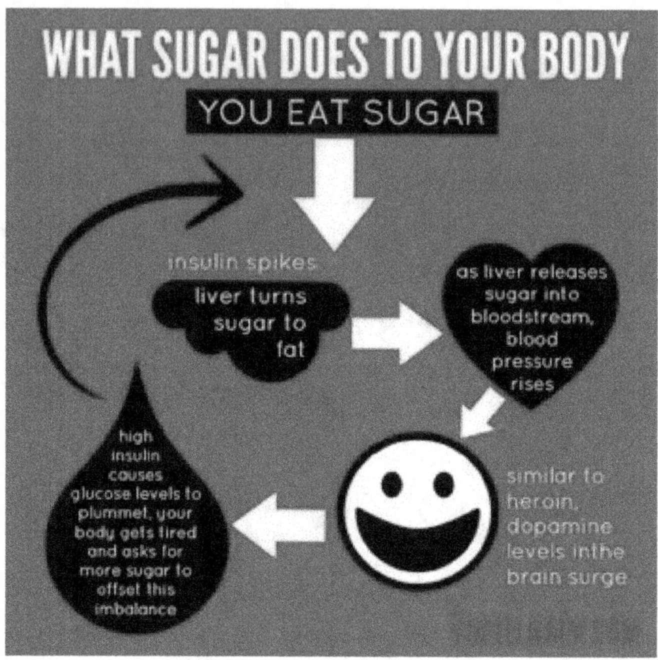

https://i.pinimg.com/736x/2e/d2/29/2ed2290964d7b73514cc8b121196cfa3--healthy-detox-detox-foods.jpg

As already mentioned lower levels of sugar in your diet can prevent the onset of diabetes and heart disease. However; sugar is also known to irritate your stomach; causing it to become inflamed.

Inflamed stomachs will provide the perfect environment for bacteria to grow. Initially you may simply experience discomfort, but this can lead to IBS, indigestion and eve ulcers.

A lower sugar intake will make you feel healthier!

2. **Filling Up**

When you get hungry the first thing most people reach for is a sugary snack. This takes the edge off your huger and gives you an instant energy boost.

Unfortunately, the effects are short-lived. You will quickly find yourself feeling hungry again and low on energy.

By reducing sugar intake and reaching for a protein rich snack you will avoid the hunger cycle created by a sugar dependency. You will also feel fuller for longer.

3. Energy

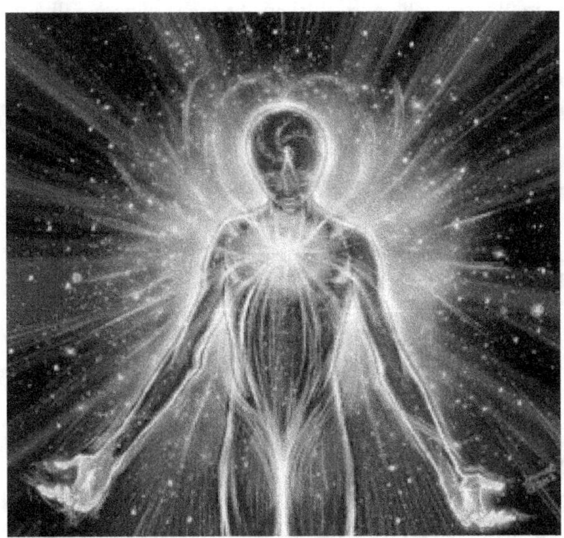

http://www.healingenergytools.com/wp-content/uploads/2016/04/Ssv5r7zNI6U_U29q1efkzsI_AAAAAAAANEk_-Tu168_W_ctI_s1600_energy_body___frequency_disease.jpg

Your energy should come from slow releasing carbs and proteins. However, most people rely on the ht provided by sugar to give them a boost throughout the day.

The result is your energy levels go up and down throughout the day. However, removing the sugar and eating healthier will allow you to have a stable supply of energy all day. You will feel more energetic than you currently do!

4. Better Moods

Excess sugar consumption causes you to feel good; this is often followed by a period of feeling low. In effect, your mood will swing from positive to negative in a short space of time.

Repeated mood swings will make it much more difficult to focus successfully on any specific project.

By detoxing and then minimizing your sugar intake you will quickly discover that your mood is more stable and generally more positive all the time.

5. Control

Once you have completed a sugar detox you will feel more in control of your body. You will no longer be subject to sugar cravings and fluctuations in your energy levels. This is not to say you will feel fantastic all the time.

But, you will be more in control of your body and more conscious about what foods you are eating. This can have a huge impact on your health in the future; helping you to stay younger looking and healthier for longer.

6. Reducing Wrinkles

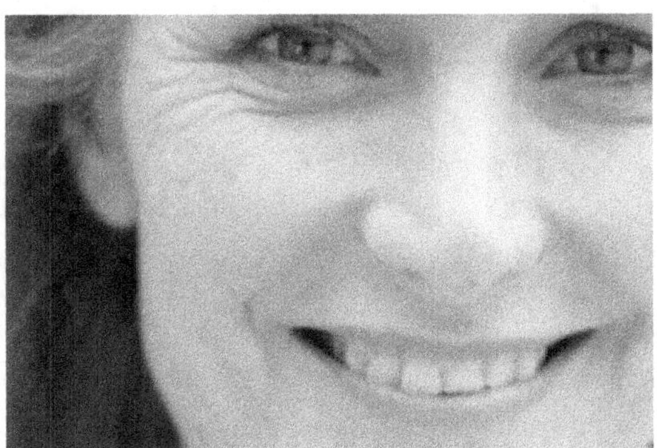

https://steptohealth.com/wp-content/uploads/2015/02/wrinkles.png

Research shows that free sugar contains a compound which when consumed causes visible damage to your skin; in the form of wrinkles.

He compound is known as glycation and, when mixed with oxygen, it causes dryness. This can cause damage on the inside of your body. On the outside it will appear as dry skin and wrinkles.

Reducing your sugar intake can actually help to eliminate these fine wrinkles.

7. Saving Money

Processed food is high in sugar, but it is also cheap to buy and generally easy to prepare. This is the main reason that most people choose to eat processed foods; convenience is valued highly in the fast paced modern world.

However, excess sugar consumption leads to a variety of health issues, from simple indigestion, to heart disease and diabetes.

The result of this is often a multitude of sick days and the need to purchase medication. In the long run, your processed food purchases will cost you more financially than purchasing ingredients and making healthy meals.

8. Sex Drive

Your sex drive is driven by hormones; the creation of which is carefully balanced by your body to ensure all your needs are met.

Unfortunately, excessive consumption of any substance can disturb your body's ability to balance hormones. Excess sugar consumption has been shown to decrease your sex drive; which is also influenced by environmental toxins and stress.

9. Set an Example

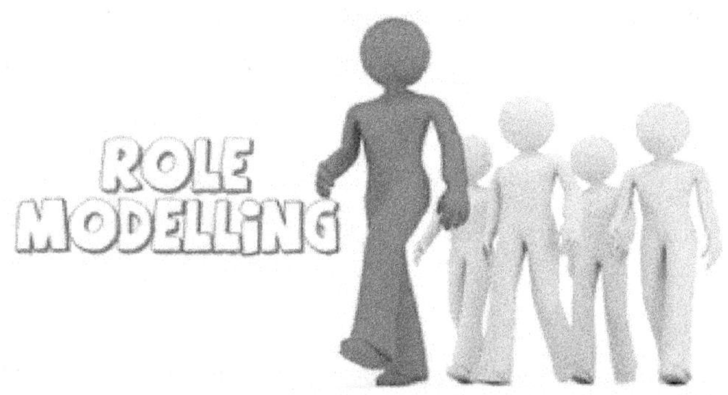

http://campuslinklive.org/wp-content/uploads/2015/02/rolemodelling.jpg

Every parent wants to give their child the best possible start in life. One of the ways to do this is to set a good example for them to follow. Consuming excessive amounts of free sugars will be detrimental to anyone's health; by reducing or

eliminating your sugar intake you can set an example which your children,
friends and even colleagues can copy.

You literally can change the world.

Conclusion

When you first discover the concept of a sugar detox you may think that it does not apply to you, you are simply not consuming too much sugar. This is especially true if you try to avoid biscuits and sweets.

However, this does not mean that you will not benefit from a sugar detox! Once you start looking at the level of sugar in everyday items of food you will be surprised at how much you are actually consuming.

When you consider this in conjunction with how little sugar the human body needs on a daily basis, you will quickly realize that the majority of people are consuming too much sugar and could benefit from a sugar detox

Detoxing offers an array of health benefits; as already discussed in this book. You will find different resources which indicate it is possible to detox in anything from 3 days to 3 months.

This guide suggests two weeks is the right timeline, there are several reasons for this:

- **Resetting the Palate**

Removing sugar and the other foods listed in this book will effectively reset your taste buds. You will appreciate the natural sweetness of food more and find that you crave sugar less; just because you can taste the natural flavors better.

- **Learn About Food**

You may also be surprised at how much you will learn about different food types; not just their sugar content.

This should motivate and inspire you into making healthier eating choices.

- **Discover Alternative Eating Options**

The desire to eat more healthily will encourage you to choose alternative food sources which can broaden your palate and provide you with an entire range of food that you may never have considered before.

Once your palate has been reset and you have passed the halfway mark of your detox, you will find that the process starts to get easier. Your energy level will be more consistent and you can enjoy trying a range of foods; as though you have never tasted them before!

A sugar detox takes a small amount of planning and very little of your time. You will need to plan your meals and your shopping trip more carefully; you will also find you are consuming less takeaways and more natural, hoe baked options.

This small amount of effort can provide you with a huge range of health benefits; providing you commit to a lifestyle that minimizes added sugar intake. This does not mean you need to eliminate it completely. As with anything in life, moderation and balance is the key to a healthy, happy life.

FREE Bonus Reminder

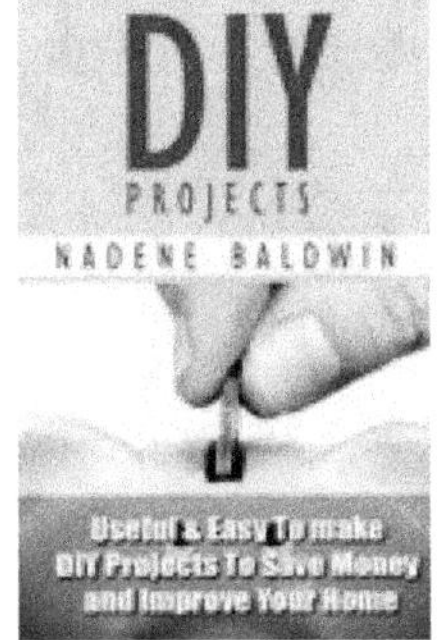

If you have not grabbed it yet, please go ahead and download your special bonus report *"DIY Projects. 13 Useful & Easy To Make DIY Projects To Save Money & Improve Your Home!"*

Simply Click the Button Below

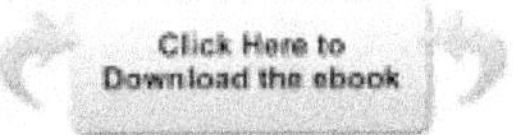

OR **Go to This Page**

http://diyhomecraft.com/free

BONUS #2: More Free & Discounted Books or Products

Do you want to receive more Free/Discounted Books or Products?

We have a mailing list where we send out our new Books or Products when they go free or with a discount on Amazon. Click on the link below to sign up for Free & Discount Book & Product Promotions.

=> Sign Up for Free & Discount Book & Product Promotions <=

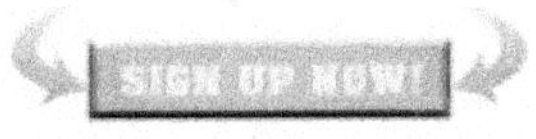

OR Go to this URL

http://zbit.ly/1WBb1Ek